GISELE BUNDCHEN

BIOGRAPHY

A Supermodel's Journey to Stardom:From Humble Beginnings to Global Icons.

Gerard Lawson

Disclaimer

This book contains information that is solely meant to be educational. Despite their best efforts to present accurate and current information, the author and publisher disclaim all expre tossed and implied representations and warranties regarding the availability, completeness, accuracy, reliability, suitability, or suitability of the content contained herein for any purpose. The publisher and the author disclaim all responsibility for any loss or harm, including without limitation, consequential or indirect loss or damage, or any loss or damage at all resulting from lost profits or data resulting from using this book.

Table of contents

INTRODUCTION

The Rise of a Supermodel

Gisele Bündchen's incredible journey from a small town in Brazil to becoming one of the world's most iconic supermodels.

Gisele Bündchen is not just a name; it's a phenomenon. From a small town in Brazil to the glittering stages of the global fashion industry, her journey is nothing short of extraordinary. This book, Gisele Bündchen: A Supermodel's Journey to Stardom.From Humble Beginnings to Global Icon, captures the story of a woman whose determination, resilience, and unique charm turned her into one of the most celebrated figures in fashion history.

Born in 1980 in the quiet town of Horizontina, Brazil, Gisele grew up in a family of modest means. She was one of six sisters, raised with values of hard work, humility, and a deep connection to nature. Little did anyone know that this tall, slender girl with striking features would go on to redefine the modeling industry and become an inspiration for millions around the world.

The story of Gisele's rise is as much about talent as it is about grit. Discovered at the age of 14 by a talent scout in a shopping mall, she was thrust into a world that was both dazzling and daunting. In an industry often defined by fleeting trends and fierce competition, Gisele stood out not just for her physical attributes but for her discipline, professionalism, and the undeniable aura she brought to every runway and photoshoot.

Her breakthrough moment came when she became the face of Victoria's Secret, earning her the title of a supermodel and making her a household name. Gisele's signature walk, often described as confident and powerful, set her apart from her peers. She brought a refreshing energy to the fashion world, which at the time was dominated by waif-like figures of the 1990s. Gisele ushered in the era of the Brazilian Bombshell, representing a new kind of beauty, strong, athletic, and unapologetically confident.

But her influence extended far beyond the runway. Gisele leveraged her platform to champion environmental causes, promote wellness, and advocate for sustainable practices in fashion. She became a symbol of what it means to use fame for a purpose, proving that beauty and substance can go hand in hand. Whether she's planting trees in the Amazon rainforest or speaking at global summits, Gisele has consistently used her voice to make a difference.

This book delves into every aspect of Gisele's life: her early struggles, her rise to fame, and the challenges she faced along the way. It also explores her personal life of her marriage to NFL superstar Tom Brady, her role as a mother, and her journey of self-discovery. Gisele is not just a supermodel; she is a businesswoman, an author, a philanthropist, and a cultural icon.

Through her story, we see the power of persistence and authenticity. Gisele's journey reminds us that even in a world obsessed with appearances, what truly matters is the person you are beneath the surface. Her ability to stay true to herself, embrace her roots, and give back to the world has solidified her legacy as more than just a pretty face. She is a force to be reckoned with.

Whether you are a fashion enthusiast, an aspiring model, or someone seeking inspiration, Gisele's story offers valuable lessons about the importance of hard work, resilience, and staying grounded. She has shown us that greatness is not just about achieving success but also about using that success to uplift others and leave the world better than you found it.

Join us as we explore the life and legacy of Gisele Bündchen, a woman who started with nothing but a dream and became a global icon. This is her story, a tale of passion, perseverance, and purpose.

CHAPTER 1: EARLY LIFE-HUMBLE BEGINNINGS IN BRAZIL

Gisele Bündchen's journey from a small town in Brazil to becoming one of the world's most recognized supermodels is a testament to her determination and the early influences that shaped her life. Born on July 20, 1980, in Horizontina, a quiet town in southern Brazil, Gisele grew up in a large family. Her parents, Vânia, a retired bank clerk, and Valdir Bündchen, a psychologist, provided a stable and supportive home environment. Gisele was the 15th child in a family of 20 siblings, which gave her a unique perspective on family dynamics, discipline, and the value of hard work.

A Family-Oriented Upbringing

Gisele's family played a central role in her development. Growing up in such a large family meant that she had to share attention and resources, which fostered a sense of independence and resilience from an early age. Although Gisele was one of the youngest in the family, her parents instilled in her the importance of education, respect, and responsibility. Her mother, Vânia, was particularly influential in encouraging Gisele's interest in beauty and fashion, but she also emphasized the importance of staying grounded.

In a family where everyone had their interests and ambitions, Gisele was encouraged to pursue her passions. Her father, Valdir, was supportive of Gisele's dreams, always motivating her to be the best version of herself. Gisele's upbringing in Horizontina, surrounded by a large, close-knit family, gave her a sense of belonging and security that helped her stay focused as she grew older. Despite the size of her family, Gisele's childhood was not one of wealth. The family lived modestly, and the emphasis was always on values rather than material possessions. This humble beginning gave Gisele the strength to face challenges later in life with resilience and perseverance.

A Small Town, Big Dreams

Growing up in Horizontina, a town with a population of only a few thousand, Gisele's world was much smaller than the glitzy fashion capitals she would one day conquer. In a town where most people worked regular jobs in agriculture or commerce, the world of fashion seemed far away. However, Gisele had big dreams. She would often browse through magazines and look at pictures of models and celebrities, imagining herself in their place. Though she was very young at the time, Gisele's natural beauty and tall, slender frame caught the attention of others.

She was an active child, always involved in sports, particularly volleyball, and she excelled at it. Gisele was not just the tall, pretty girl in town; she was also strong, determined, and athletic. These qualities shaped her character and helped her navigate the challenges she would face as she pursued a career in modeling. But as much as she enjoyed sports, she also had an innate interest in fashion, and this desire to step into the world of modeling was something that remained with her.

Gisele's dreams began to feel attainable when, at the age of 13, she enrolled in a modeling course in the nearby city of Porto Alegre. This was her first step into the world of fashion, and although it was a modest beginning, it set the stage for the incredible career she would eventually have. During this time, Gisele also worked on her confidence, learning the importance of posture, walking, and developing a strong sense of self.

Her family remained a key support system, helping her navigate these early experiences and ensuring she stayed true to her values.

The Influence of Her Brazilian Heritage

As Gisele developed her sense of identity, her Brazilian heritage played a significant role in shaping the woman she would become. Brazil is known for its rich culture, colorful festivals, and appreciation for beauty, all of which had a lasting influence on Gisele. Growing up in Brazil, Gisele was surrounded by a culture that celebrated both natural beauty and individual expression.

Brazilian beauty standards, which embrace a diverse range of physical appearances, allowed

Gisele to feel comfortable with her looks. Her naturally long, golden hair and strong, athletic build became part of the signature look that would later make her a global icon. Gisele's embrace of her heritage and physical traits helped her stand out in the modeling industry, where tall, slim, and symmetrical features are often the norm.

Beyond her physical appearance, Gisele's Brazilian roots instilled in her a love for nature and a deep sense of connection to the environment. Growing up in a country with such vast natural beauty, Gisele developed an appreciation for sustainability and the importance of preserving the planet. This would later shape her commitment to environmental activism as she became a well-known figure in the fashion industry.

Her First Steps Toward Modeling

As Gisele's passion for fashion and modeling grew, she took her first concrete step toward turning her dream into reality. At 14, she attended a modeling competition in São Paulo, where her potential was immediately recognized. While she didn't win the competition, her talent was evident, and she caught the attention of several important figures in the industry. It wasn't long before Gisele's career began to take shape, as she received offers to model for local fashion designers and participate in fashion shows.

However, breaking into the modeling world wasn't easy, especially for someone coming from a small town in Brazil. The world of high fashion, filled with glamorous and competitive environments, was vastly different from Gisele's simple upbringing. Still, she remained determined, using her family's support as a foundation for her success. They encouraged her to take the opportunities that came her way, even if they meant leaving her hometown and traveling to far-off cities.

The Role of Education and Discipline

Although Gisele's career path shifted towards modeling, her education remained a priority. Gisele attended school until she was about 16, maintaining a strong academic record. She credits her education for helping her build the discipline and focus needed to succeed in her career. Even though modeling became her main focus, Gisele believes that her academic experiences and the values she learned in school contributed to her success.

Her family also emphasized the importance of self-discipline. Gisele was taught to work hard for everything she achieved, and this mindset became ingrained in her. As her modeling career grew, Gisele found herself balancing her work commitments with the need for personal growth and development. She never lost sight of the lessons learned during her upbringing in Horizontina, and these lessons have played an essential role in her ability to overcome challenges in the competitive world of fashion.

A Humble Beginning, A Global Future

Gisele Bündchen's early life in Horizontina, Brazil, was marked by humble beginnings, a strong family unit, and the development of a dream. Her journey from a small town to international fame is a story of resilience, ambition, and the power of believing in one's potential. As Gisele's career took off, she carried with her the values, lessons, and strength instilled in her by her family and the small Brazilian town that shaped her.

CHAPTER 2: THE DISCOVERY- A LIFE-CHANGING MOMENT

Gisele Bündchen's life changed dramatically when she was discovered as a teenager in Brazil. This pivotal moment marked the beginning of her extraordinary career in modeling, setting her on a path to becoming one of the most famous and successful supermodels in the world. Her story is one of chance, perseverance, and the perfect timing that brought her into the global spotlight.

A Teenager with Big Dreams

Before Gisele's big break, she was just a 13-year-old girl living in Horizontina, a small town in southern Brazil. She had always been tall for her age, with long legs and a distinctive, natural beauty that made her stand out. However, Gisele was not yet aware of the world of high fashion. She spent most of her time playing sports and hanging out with friends, dreaming of something bigger but not sure how to get there. Her family supported her in every way, but they did not initially encourage her to pursue a career in modeling, as they were focused on her education and well-being.

At the time, Gisele had no idea that the world of fashion was just around the corner. Her family had never been involved in the fashion industry, and the idea of becoming a model seemed far-fetched. Still, Gisele was a determined young woman, and she had an inner drive that pushed her to seek new opportunities. Her athleticism and natural beauty were the first things people noticed about her, but it would take someone with a keen eye to see her potential as a model.

The Discovery: A Fortuitous Encounter

Gisele's life would change forever when she attended a modeling course in Porto Alegre, a larger city in southern Brazil. It was here, in 1994, that Gisele's potential was first recognized by an industry insider. While she was participating in the course, a modeling agent named Elite Model Management was impressed by her height, her graceful posture, and the raw beauty that radiated from her. He saw something in Gisele that set her apart from the other students in the course. Gisele was just 14 years old at the time, and while she was still growing into herself, the agent immediately saw the star quality that would make her stand out in the competitive world of fashion.

This discovery was nothing short of a lucky break, as Gisele had never considered modeling as a serious career. The agent was captivated by her potential, offering her the chance to join Elite Model Management in São Paulo. At the time, Gisele was hesitant to leave her small town and embark on a career she knew little about. She had little experience in modeling and didn't fully understand the opportunities that were opening up to her. However, her family supported her decision to take a chance on this new path, and after much encouragement, she agreed to leap.

The First Steps-Learning the Ropes

When Gisele arrived in São Paulo, she was faced with a completely new world. The bustling, fast-paced city was far from her quiet hometown in Horizontina. She began to learn about the industry, its expectations, and the hard work required to succeed. Gisele quickly realized that modeling was not as glamorous as she had imagined. It involved long hours, constant competition, and an overwhelming need for discipline and professionalism.

At first, Gisele's experience in São Paulo was a challenging one. She faced rejection and had to work hard to prove herself in an industry that often favored those with more experience. Many established models looked more polished and had already gained recognition in the fashion world. Gisele had to work on perfecting her walk, her facial expressions, and how to present herself in front of the camera. She also had to learn how to handle criticism and rejection, which are common in the modeling world.

However, Gisele was determined to succeed. Her perseverance and strong work ethic helped her stay focused. She took on smaller jobs to gain experience, and slowly but surely, her efforts began to pay off. After a few months, she started getting noticed by more designers, photographers, and agencies. Her natural beauty, combined with her dedication to improving her craft, began to set her apart from other models in São Paulo.

The Turning Point- A Fashion Show Breakthrough

Gisele's breakthrough moment came in 1996 when she was chosen to walk in a major fashion show. It was a huge opportunity for the young model, and it was her chance to prove that she could shine on the international stage. During the show, Gisele stood out for her grace and poise on the runway. She captured the attention of fashion industry professionals, photographers, and designers, all of whom saw her as a rising star.

The show was a pivotal moment for Gisele because it proved that she was not just another aspiring model; she had the potential to be a major player in the industry. Following the fashion show, Gisele began to receive more attention from high-profile designers and photographers. Her distinct look a mix of Brazilian beauty with European influence made her a unique presence in the fashion world.

Soon after, she started booking more prominent gigs, working with top designers and appearing in major campaigns. Gisele's career began to take off, and she quickly gained a reputation for being one of the most sought-after models in the industry. Within just a few years, Gisele became the face of high-fashion brands like Versace, Dolce & Gabbana, and Valentino. Her star was rising, and it was clear that she was destined for greatness.

A Journey of Perseverance

Gisele's discovery was just the beginning of her journey. While her path to success seemed almost serendipitous, it was also shaped by her hard work, dedication, and resilience. Even though Gisele faced many challenges in the early stages of her career, she never gave up. She continued to learn, grow, and improve, constantly refining her craft.

The modeling industry is incredibly competitive, and countless aspiring models are vying for the same opportunities. Gisele's success was not just due to her beauty; it was the result of her relentless drive and willingness to work hard every single day.

Her discovery as a teenager was indeed a life-changing moment, but it was only the beginning of a career that would span decades and make her one of the most iconic supermodels of all time. Her journey is a powerful reminder that sometimes, life-changing opportunities come from unexpected places, and with the right combination of talent, determination, and luck, dreams can come true.

CHAPTER 3: BREAKING INTO THE FASHION WORLD-STRUGGLES AND TRIUMPHS

Gisele Bündchen's journey into the fashion world was not a smooth and effortless path, but one filled with hard work, determination, and overcoming many obstacles. Her early years as a model were a series of challenges, from rejection to learning how to navigate the highly competitive and often demanding world of high fashion. Yet, these struggles were crucial in shaping Gisele into the global icon she would become.

Facing Rejection and Doubts

When Gisele first entered the modeling industry, she encountered a great deal of rejection. Despite her natural beauty and striking looks, she wasn't immediately accepted by the fashion world. It was difficult to get noticed, especially in an industry where so many other aspiring models were trying to make a name for themselves. At the time, many models were praised for their slim figures, and Gisele was often told that she was too tall, too curvy, and even too different from the "ideal" look.

In the early stages of her career, Gisele faced many casting rejections. She was told that she didn't fit the conventional model standards that were prevalent at the time. The fashion world was very much focused on a particular body type, and Gisele's physical appearance, while undeniably beautiful, didn't always align with that narrow standard. This led to self-doubt and uncertainty, but rather than giving up, Gisele used the feedback to fuel her determination.

Building Confidence and Skills

After her initial struggles, Gisele understood that to succeed in the modeling industry, she would need to build her confidence and work hard to improve her skills. She committed herself to learning everything she could about modeling and fashion. This meant working on her runway walk, mastering facial expressions, and understanding how to convey different emotions through photographs.

In the beginning, she was often nervous and unsure in front of the camera. Modeling wasn't just about looking beautiful; it was also about understanding the art of posing, expressing emotion, and adapting to different styles. Gisele spent time perfecting these techniques, and over time, she gained more confidence. She learned that it wasn't enough just to be beautiful. She needed to show personality, versatility, and professionalism.

This hard work began to pay off as Gisele started landing more jobs. The fashion industry began to notice her unique look, and she started to book more runway shows, magazine covers, and advertising campaigns. Though she still faced challenges, her growing experience and improving skills gave her the resilience she needed to push forward.

The Big Break- A Turning Point

The turning point in Gisele's career came when she secured a major contract with the prestigious designer, Alexander McQueen, and booked high-profile shows. These opportunities opened doors for Gisele that she could never have imagined in her early years. The fashion industry began to take her seriously, and her name started to appear in the media.

One of the most defining moments in her career was when Gisele was invited to walk in the Victoria's Secret Fashion Show in 1999. This was a game-changer for Gisele. Victoria's Secret, at the time, was one of the most well-known and widely televised fashion events, and being chosen to participate in such a prominent show brought Gisele's career to the forefront. Not only did it introduce her to a massive global audience, but it also solidified her position as one of the top models in the world.

It was during this period that Gisele began to find her signature style a combination of athleticism, grace, and sensuality, which set her apart from many of her peers. She quickly became the face of major campaigns, including campaigns for brands like Versace, Dolce & Gabbana, and Valentino. Gisele's ability to bring both elegance and strength to her work allowed her to stand out in a crowded industry.

Challenges with Media and Public Perception

Though Gisele's career was on an upward trajectory, she continued to face challenges, especially with the media. As one of the world's most famous models, Gisele was constantly in the public eye, and the pressure to maintain a certain image weighed heavily on her. The media often scrutinized her personal life, her appearance, and even her opinions on various topics. This level of attention was overwhelming at times, especially for someone who was still growing into adulthood and learning how to handle fame.

Despite these pressures, Gisele remained focused on her work. She knew that the public's perception of her could fluctuate, but she kept a clear sense of purpose. Rather than letting the media's scrutiny affect her, she focused on what she could control her professionalism and her passion for her craft. Over time, this allowed her to create a brand for herself that was strong and independent, based not just on her looks but also on her dedication and work ethic.

A Rising Star

By the early 2000s, Gisele had cemented herself as one of the top models in the world. She had overcome the struggles of rejection, self-doubt, and industry pressures to become a force in the fashion world. Gisele's rise was a direct result of her perseverance, the lessons she learned from her early challenges, and her ability to embrace her unique qualities. She had finally reached a place in her career where her name was synonymous with fashion and beauty, and she was being recognized as one of the greatest supermodels of her generation.

Her work with high-profile designers, her presence in international campaigns, and her iconic runway moments solidified her place in fashion history. Gisele had become a global household name. But what was most impressive about her rise was not just her ability to succeed in a competitive industry, but how she remained grounded despite her fame.

Legacy of Resilience

Looking back on Gisele's early years, her success is a testament to resilience. She faced many hurdles and challenges that could have easily led her to quit, but she pushed through them, learning and growing with each experience. The lessons she learned during her struggles helped to shape the model she became, and today, she stands as an inspiration to many young women and aspiring models who face similar challenges.

Gisele's story proves that even in an industry where rejection is common and the competition is fierce, determination, self-belief, and hard work can lead to incredible success. The struggles she overcame early in her career were not obstacles, but stepping stones on her journey to becoming one of the most influential supermodels in history.

CHAPTER 4: VICTORIA'S SECRET-A SUPERMODEL IS BORN

Gisele Bündchen's rise to supermodel status was significantly shaped by her collaboration with Victoria's Secret, a brand that would become synonymous with her name and cement her place in the fashion world. Her partnership with the iconic lingerie brand not only launched her into global fame but also played a pivotal role in reshaping the modeling industry. This collaboration marked the moment Gisele transitioned from a well-known model to a household name.

The Beginning of the Partnership

Gisele's first encounter with Victoria's Secret came in 1999 when she was still building her reputation as a model. Victoria's Secret, known for its glamorous runway shows and powerful marketing campaigns, was looking for fresh faces to represent the brand. At the time, the brand's roster of models included some of the most famous names in the fashion industry, such as Tyra Banks and Heidi Klum. However, the brand was looking for something new. someone who could capture the attention of a global audience.

Gisele, with her tall, athletic frame and unique beauty, caught the eye of the brand's executives. Her look stood out as different from the typical "cookie-cutter" models that dominated the fashion world at the time. In 1999, she walked in her first Victoria's Secret Fashion Show, and from that moment, everything began to change.

The Iconic Victoria's Secret Fashion Show

The Victoria's Secret Fashion Show, known for its glitz, glamour, and extravagant themes, was a key moment in Gisele's journey to superstardom. With each show, the brand showcased top models, known as "Angels," walking the runway in elaborate lingerie, wings, and other iconic costumes. The show was broadcast globally, attracting millions of viewers, and for a model, it was a golden opportunity to be seen by an enormous audience.

Gisele's first appearance on the Victoria's Secret runway was a breakthrough. She captivated the audience with her presence, grace, and confident walk, which set her apart from her peers. She wasn't just another pretty face in lingerie. She exuded strength, sensuality, and elegance, a combination that helped her stand out among the other Angels. As she continued to walk in the show over the next few years, Gisele's popularity grew exponentially. Her striking beauty, combined with her ability to embody both strength and femininity, resonated with viewers and photographers alike.

By 2000, Gisele had become a regular in the Victoria's Secret Fashion Show, and her presence was soon synonymous with the brand's image. The more she appeared on the runway, the more the public took notice. As a result, she began landing more high-profile contracts, both with Victoria's Secret and other global brands.

Becoming the Face of Victoria's Secret

As Gisele's career soared, so did her partnership with Victoria's Secret. By 2000, she became one of the most recognized faces of the brand. Her involvement with Victoria's Secret was more than just walking in the annual shows. She was featured in some of the brand's most prominent advertising campaigns, from print ads to television commercials. She soon became one of the brand's top models and was given the coveted title of "Angel."

Victoria's Secret helped Gisele break into mainstream culture. The campaigns she appeared in became iconic, and she started to be recognized not only as a model but as a fashion personality. Her face appeared on billboards, in magazines, and in television commercials worldwide. She was no longer just a model in the industry; she was a star. This visibility also helped her transition from a niche figure in fashion to a global name that transcended the world of modeling. Gisele's association with Victoria's Secret helped solidify her brand as a top-tier, high-fashion supermodel.

Impact on Gisele's Global Fame

Victoria's Secret provided Gisele with a platform like no other. The brand's fashion shows, which were broadcast to millions of viewers, turned the annual event into an entertainment spectacle. Gisele's presence on that stage allowed her to reach a broad, diverse audience, many of whom were not typically interested in fashion but tuned in for the glamour, excitement, and star-studded event. Through her appearances, Gisele's popularity spread far beyond the fashion world, making her a household name.

In addition to her appearances on the runway, Gisele's work with Victoria's Secret also included high-fashion photoshoots and ad campaigns. She quickly became the face of the brand's lingerie, swimwear, and fragrance lines. Her stunning looks and magnetic presence in these advertisements helped solidify her as one of the most influential models of her time.

By the early 2000s, Gisele was no longer just a part of the Victoria's Secret roster. She had become one of its key figures. She was one of the brand's most prominent Angels, and her association with the company was instrumental in her rise to global fame. Gisele had achieved the kind of success that many models dream of but few ever attain.

Changing the Face of the Fashion Industry

Gisele's collaboration with Victoria's Secret did more than just propel her career; it also contributed to changing beauty standards in the fashion world. Before her rise, the fashion industry was dominated by very slim, often underweight models. Gisele, with her athletic build, strong body, and healthy appearance, represented a new standard of beauty. She helped redefine what it meant to be a successful model at a time when the industry's definition of beauty was shifting.

Her collaboration with Victoria's Secret helped highlight the power of diversity in modeling and brought attention to the importance of a more inclusive vision of beauty. This was a significant moment in the modeling world, where other brands and designers started to recognize that there was a wider variety of beauty that could be celebrated. Gisele's ability to effortlessly blend strength, elegance, and sensuality helped to break down outdated stereotypes and allowed for a more dynamic and varied range of models to thrive in the fashion industry.

The Legacy of Victoria's Secret

Gisele's partnership with Victoria's Secret not only shaped her career but also left an indelible mark on the fashion industry. Her time with the brand solidified her as one of the greatest supermodels of all time. It was during her collaboration with Victoria's Secret that she became synonymous with the word "supermodel," a title that few could ever claim.

Through her work with the brand, Gisele gained more than just fame. She gained the kind of influence that few models in history have held. Her global popularity, her role as an icon of beauty and strength, and her dedication to her craft ensured that her name would be forever linked with the Victoria's Secret brand. More than that, she helped elevate the brand to new heights, turning it into a cultural phenomenon.

Her time with Victoria's Secret remains one of the defining moments of her career, and it will continue to be remembered as the time when Gisele Bündchen truly became a global household name.

CHAPTER 5: REVOLUTIONIZING BEAUTY STANDARDS-GISELE'S IMPACT ON FASHION

Gisele Bündchen's entry into the fashion industry came at a time when beauty ideals were shifting. For decades, the standard model body was thin, often fragile-looking, and lacking in muscular tone. Models were expected to embody a certain, almost ethereal quality. However, Gisele, with her athletic build, strong presence, and healthy curves, helped challenge and redefine these ideals. She became an icon not just because of her beauty but because of the way she represented a new, more inclusive vision of what beauty could look like.

Breaking Away from Traditional Beauty Norms

When Gisele began her career in the late 1990s, the fashion industry was still largely influenced by the grunge and minimalistic looks that defined the early part of the decade. The models who were successful in the 1990s, such as Kate Moss, embodied the "heroin chic" look a tall, very slim frame that lacked the curves and muscle tone seen in previous decades. These models were often celebrated for their waif-like, almost fragile appearance. Gisele, however, was different.

Her athletic build, strong jawline, and healthy curves marked a clear departure from the models of that era. Gisele's body type was more reminiscent of the traditional "Brazilian bombshell".A woman who was strong, confident, and naturally curvy. She was a fresh face in an industry that was beginning to recognize the need for a broader, more diverse representation of beauty. While many models were being pushed into one mold, Gisele brought a new energy to the fashion scene, and she quickly became one of the most sought-after models in the world.

The Brazilian Bombshell

Gisele's look became an iconic representation of what was often called the "Brazilian bombshell".A term that alluded to a specific combination of femininity, strength, and sensuality. Brazilian women, known for their curves and confidence, had long been celebrated in global beauty standards, and Gisele embodied this ideal perfectly. Her long legs, toned body, and full lips made her stand out from the rest. She became a symbol of health and strength, proving that a model did not have to be overly thin to be considered beautiful or successful.

Her stunning looks represented a shift away from the ultra-thin aesthetic that had dominated the fashion industry in the past. Gisele's features her athletic build, her glowing skin, and her sharp yet approachable features became a new kind of standard. This marked the beginning of a new era in modeling, one that allowed for a broader interpretation of beauty and, ultimately, more opportunities for models with diverse body types and backgrounds.

Challenging Beauty Ideals in the Fashion Industry

Before Gisele's rise, few models could be considered muscular or visibly healthy. Instead, the fashion industry celebrated models who were often extremely thin, sometimes to the point of unhealthy levels. Gisele, however, was different. She embraced her curves and her toned, muscular physique, which became part of her signature look. Her body was strong yet feminine, a combination that defied the conventional expectations of models at the time.

As her career progressed, Gisele became one of the first major models to publicly embrace and celebrate her healthy lifestyle. She wasn't just a pretty face on the runway; she was a symbol of what it meant to take care of one's body and to embrace a more natural, attainable form of beauty. Her athleticism became a core part of her identity, and it became clear that her beauty was not just about how she looked, but about how she carried herself. Her strength, confidence, and focus on well-being became an essential part of her appeal.

Gisele's rise to stardom played a key role in pushing the fashion industry to acknowledge and embrace different types of beauty. Her broad shoulders, sculpted legs, and naturally healthy curves helped to open the door for models who did not fit the traditional, ultra-thin mold. Over time, Gisele's presence in the industry helped break down rigid beauty standards and made it clear that a more diverse, inclusive definition of beauty was not only possible but necessary.

The Evolution of Beauty in the 21st Century

The success of Gisele and other models who embodied a more athletic, fuller-bodied aesthetic marked the beginning of a significant change in the industry. Gisele helped prove that beauty was not defined by a single, narrow ideal. Her fame and influence allowed her to bring a new, refreshing approach to modeling, one that celebrated strength, health, and confidence.

As Gisele's career progressed, the fashion industry began to take notice of her impact. Other brands and designers started to embrace models with more muscular builds and curvier figures. This change didn't happen overnight, but Gisele's visibility in the fashion world made it easier for future models who didn't fit the "traditional" mold to find success. She showed the world that beauty could be diverse and could be defined by strength, vitality, and confidence, rather than just by size or shape.

The influence of Gisele and other models who challenged traditional beauty norms cannot be overstated. She helped shift the conversation about body image in fashion, proving that beauty could look different on everyone and still be powerful and captivating.

A Lasting Impact on Fashion and Beauty

Gisele's role in revolutionizing beauty standards was not only about her physical appearance but also about how she carried herself as a professional. Her dedication to fitness, health, and well-being made her a role model for many, and her advocacy for a more inclusive idea of beauty helped change the way the fashion industry approached models and beauty.

Through her success, Gisele demonstrated that beauty is not just about fitting into a certain box, but about embracing individuality and confidence. Her partnership with top brands, her unforgettable runway walks, and her consistent message of health and strength made her a force to be reckoned with in the fashion world.

Even today, Gisele's impact is still felt. The fashion industry continues to evolve, and the inclusivity she championed is becoming more widespread. Models of different body types, backgrounds, and ethnicities are now represented in fashion campaigns, magazine covers, and runway shows, thanks in part to Gisele's groundbreaking work. She helped shift the beauty ideal from a one-dimensional standard to a more nuanced and diverse vision.

Gisele's influence was far-reaching and transformative. She proved that beauty could be strong, natural, and healthy and in doing so, she set a new standard for models to aspire to. Through her iconic looks and trailblazing career, she became more than just a supermodel. She became a symbol of a new, more inclusive approach to beauty.

CHAPTER 6: Iconic Runway Moments and Designer Collaborations

Gisele Bündchen's career has been marked by numerous iconic runway moments that have solidified her place as one of the most celebrated supermodels in history. Her work with top designers, unforgettable runway walks, and her undeniable presence on the catwalk have left an indelible mark on the fashion industry. Over the years, Gisele has partnered with some of the most renowned designers, shaping not just fashion trends, but also the future of the runway itself.

The Early Runway Moments-Breaking Into High Fashion

Gisele's first steps into the world of runway shows were an important beginning to her career. She made her debut in 1997 at New York Fashion Week, quickly catching the attention of top designers. At that time, the fashion industry was dominated by a handful of prominent models, and breaking into this elite space was no small feat. However, Gisele's confidence, striking features, and ability to walk the runway with effortless grace set her apart from the crowd.

Her first big break came when she walked for high-end designers like Alexander McQueen, Valentino, and Dolce & Gabbana. These shows marked the beginning of her transformation into a global supermodel. Gisele was not just another face on the runway; her presence commanded attention. With every stride, she brought a unique energy, which was a perfect fit for the extravagant and high-fashion shows of the late 1990s and early 2000s. Her ability to convey emotion and attitude with each step contributed to her rapid rise in the modeling world.

Collaborations with Top Designers

Gisele's career flourished as she worked with some of the biggest names in fashion. Her partnerships with designers like Tom Ford,

Chanel's Karl Lagerfeld, and Versace's Donatella Versace created unforgettable runway moments. These collaborations helped shape her as a muse for some of the most celebrated collections of the time.

One of the most notable moments came when Gisele walked in the iconic Versace runway show in 2000. The show featured her in a shimmering gold gown, with her long hair flowing behind her, becoming one of the standout moments of the season. It was a defining moment in her career, as she helped bring Versace's bold, sensual vision to life with her presence.

Another memorable collaboration was with Chanel's Karl Lagerfeld. Gisele's partnership with Lagerfeld was a powerful one, as the

designer saw in her the perfect embodiment of
Chanel's timeless elegance and modern
sensuality. Her walk-in Chanel's haute couture
shows brought her to the forefront of fashion's
elite, further cementing her status as one of the
industry's most sought-after models. Lagerfeld,
known for his exacting standards, was a major
influence in shaping Gisele's approach to
fashion and runway shows. She was often
chosen to showcase his most intricate designs,
thanks to her innate ability to bring his creations
to life.

Victoria's Secret Fashion Show-A Defining Moment in Gisele's Career

While Gisele's collaborations with high-end
designers were pivotal to her success, one of the

most important moments of her career came with her involvement in the Victoria's Secret Fashion Show. Starting in 1999, Gisele became one of the most prominent Angels, solidifying her place as one of the world's most iconic supermodels. Her walks down the runway during these events were electric, as she exuded confidence and charisma in every show.

The Victoria's Secret Fashion Show became a global event, and Gisele was often the star of the spectacle. In 2000, she opened the show in a sexy, feathery costume that became one of the most memorable outfits in the brand's history. Her chemistry with the audience and her stunning ability to showcase the brand's glamorous lingerie made her one of the most celebrated models in the fashion world at the time.

Her association with Victoria's Secret also helped her transition into becoming not just a runway model, but a global personality. As the brand became more popular, so did Gisele. She was able to reach millions of people worldwide, further enhancing her impact on the fashion industry.

Walking for Haute Couture: Paris Fashion Week

Paris Fashion Week has always been a highlight for the world's top models, and Gisele was no exception. She graced the runways of some of the most exclusive haute couture shows in Paris, walking for iconic designers like Christian Dior, Givenchy, and Balenciaga. Her elegance and poise made her a standout on the runways of

Paris, and her ability to transition from high fashion to everyday glamour made her a favorite of both designers and the fashion media.

One of Gisele's most memorable haute couture moments was during the 2004 Dior show. The collection, designed by John Galliano, was dramatic and extravagant, and Gisele's portrayal of the haute couture designs showcased her versatility. She wore a stunning black gown, combining both strength and sensuality, which captured the spirit of the collection. Her ability to showcase Dior's intricate designs with precision and grace made her a muse for Galliano, who saw in her a model that could bring his wild visions to life.

Gisele as a Fashion Icon Beyond the Runway

While Gisele's runway moments with top designers were integral to her career, her influence extended far beyond just walking in shows. Over the years, she became a global fashion icon, embodying the best of luxury fashion. Her collaborations with famous brands like Louis Vuitton, Dolce & Gabbana, and Stuart Weitzman elevated her from being just a model to a worldwide symbol of beauty, style, and sophistication.

Her ability to seamlessly shift between commercial and high fashion was one of her defining traits. In her advertisements for luxury brands, Gisele portrayed an image of elegance and confidence. Yet, at the same time, she also embraced her role as a relatable figure through campaigns that reached broader, more mainstream audiences. Gisele's versatility allowed her to remain relevant in a constantly evolving industry, and her work with top designers cemented her position as one of the most recognizable faces in fashion.

Gisele's Influence on the Next Generation of Models

Gisele's runway moments and collaborations with designers had a profound impact on the modeling industry. She became a trailblazer for future generations of models, setting a new standard for what a supermodel could be. Gisele's ability to effortlessly transition between high-end fashion and commercial appeal made her an inspiration for countless aspiring models who sought to emulate her success.

In addition, Gisele's runway moments were not just about the clothes or the designers. They were about the presence she brought to the stage. Her ability to command attention with her charisma, elegance, and confidence transformed the runway experience for both designers and audiences. Today, many models look to Gisele's career as a roadmap for success in the fashion industry, and her influence is felt in the work of models who are breaking barriers and pushing boundaries in the industry.

A Lasting Legacy

Gisele Bündchen's iconic runway moments and collaborations with top designers have solidified her status as one of the most influential figures in the fashion industry. Her ability to embody the vision of some of the world's most prestigious designers, coupled with her impeccable style and presence, has made her a fashion icon whose legacy will be remembered for years to come. Gisele's impact on the runway, the brands she worked with, and the models who followed in her footsteps are undeniable. She will always be celebrated for her role in revolutionizing the fashion world.

CHAPTER 7: EXPANDING HORIZONS- GISELE'S VENTURES BEYOND MODELING

Gisele Bündchen's success as one of the world's most famous supermodels has not confined her to just the runway. Over the years, she has expanded her career into various fields, showcasing her versatility and creativity in ways that go beyond modeling. With her natural beauty, strong presence, and entrepreneurial spirit, Gisele has made significant strides in acting, writing, and several other creative pursuits. These ventures have allowed her to explore new facets of her personality, grow her influence, and continue to inspire others beyond the world of fashion.

Acting Career

In addition to her modeling career, Gisele explored acting, making a few notable appearances in films and television shows. While she is primarily known for her work on the runway, her natural charm and screen presence made her a good fit for roles in the entertainment industry. She made her film debut in the 2004 movie The Devil Wears Prada, which became a huge hit and a classic in the fashion world. Although her role was relatively small, it marked the beginning of her journey into acting. She portrayed a model who shares the screen with the film's lead, Meryl Streep, who plays a powerful fashion editor. This opportunity allowed Gisele to showcase her acting skills and opened the door for more roles in Hollywood.

Gisele's involvement in acting wasn't limited to The Devil Wears Prada. She appeared in several other films, including the 2006 film Taxi, starring alongside Queen Latifah and Jimmy Fallon. In Taxi, Gisele played herself, appearing in a scene where she competed in a race against other drivers. Though these acting roles were relatively light, they gave Gisele the chance to explore another side of her career and establish her presence in Hollywood. Her work in film may have been limited, but it still played an important role in expanding her brand and increasing her appeal to new audiences beyond the fashion world.

Writing and Publishing

As Gisele continued to build her career, she also ventured into the world of writing. Her literary work reflects her deep passion for wellness, sustainability, and her journey. In 2018, Gisele released her memoir, Lessons: My Path to a Meaningful Life, which quickly became a bestseller. In the book, Gisele shares her life story in great detail, from her early years in Brazil to her rise in the fashion world and the challenges she faced along the way. The memoir is an introspective account of her journey, highlighting her personal growth, struggles, and the lessons she has learned throughout her life.

The book explores topics that are deeply important to Gisele, including mental health, self-esteem, and balancing a successful career with a fulfilling personal life. Through her writing, Gisele opened up about the pressures she faced as a supermodel, revealing the behind-the-scenes aspects of the fashion industry that are rarely talked about. She also discusses her commitment to environmental causes and sustainability, offering insights into how she incorporates these values into her personal and professional life. Lessons were widely praised for its honest and inspiring message, and it further established Gisele as a role model for women around the world. The memoir not only gave readers a glimpse into her life but also highlighted her commitment to personal growth and her desire to inspire others.

Environmental Advocacy and Entrepreneurship

While acting and writing allowed Gisele to explore her creative side, her true passion outside of modeling lies in her dedication to environmental causes and sustainability. Over the years, Gisele has become an influential advocate for the planet, using her platform to raise awareness about climate change, deforestation, and the importance of living a sustainable life. She has worked with several environmental organizations, including the United Nations Environment Programme, to help promote eco-friendly practices and raise awareness about the pressing issues facing the Earth.

One of the ways Gisele has combined her love for the environment with her entrepreneurial spirit is through her business ventures. She has launched several initiatives that focus on sustainability and promoting a healthier, more eco-conscious lifestyle. In 2018, Gisele co-founded a skincare line called Sejaa Pure Skincare, which emphasizes natural and sustainable ingredients. The line was created to offer high-quality skincare products while minimizing the impact on the environment. Gisele's passion for natural beauty products and her commitment to sustainability have made this venture particularly special, as it reflects her values and dedication to promoting a more eco-friendly lifestyle.

Gisele has also invested in other businesses and projects that align with her beliefs in sustainability and social responsibility. She has been involved in initiatives that focus on clean energy, renewable resources, and environmental conservation. Through these ventures, she continues to prove that her influence goes far beyond modeling and that she is committed to creating a positive impact in the world. Her entrepreneurial ventures have been successful, and they reflect her desire to contribute to a better future for the planet.

Philanthropy and Social Impact

Gisele has always been passionate about giving back to the community and using her platform to support causes that are important to her. Throughout her career, she has been involved in various philanthropic endeavors, particularly in the areas of education, health, and the environment. Gisele has worked closely with organizations such as the Red Cross, Doctors Without Borders, and the Rainforest Alliance, contributing both her time and resources to help make a positive difference in the world.

In 2009, Gisele was named a Goodwill Ambassador for the United Nations Environment Programme, where she used her celebrity status to raise awareness about environmental issues and advocate for sustainable practices. She has also been involved in efforts to protect the Amazon rainforest, working with organizations dedicated to preserving the environment in Brazil. Gisele's charitable efforts extend beyond just donating money; she actively participates in campaigns and projects that aim to make lasting social and environmental changes.

Through her philanthropic work, Gisele has shown that her influence as a model goes far beyond the fashion industry. She has used her platform to address some of the world's most pressing issues, including climate change and the need for greater environmental conservation. Her dedication to social causes has inspired countless individuals, encouraging them to become more mindful of the planet and to take action to create a positive change.

Beyond the Runway: A Lasting Legacy

Gisele's ventures beyond modeling are a testament to her ability to evolve and grow as a person. While she will always be remembered as one of the greatest supermodels of all time, her work in acting, writing, entrepreneurship, and philanthropy shows that she is much more than just a fashion icon. Gisele has used her platform and success to make a real impact in the world, and her ability to expand her horizons in such diverse ways has solidified her legacy as a multifaceted and influential public figure.

Her ventures beyond modeling demonstrate that Gisele is a woman who is constantly pushing herself to explore new avenues, challenge herself, and use her success for the greater good. Whether it's through her business ventures, environmental advocacy, or philanthropic work, Gisele has proven that her influence extends far beyond the runway, and she continues to inspire people across the world to pursue their passions and make a positive impact on the planet. Through her dedication to sustainability, creativity, and giving back, Gisele Bündchen's

legacy will continue to inspire future
generations.

CHAPTER 8: ENVIRONMENTAL ACTIVISM-A VOICE FOR THE PLANET

Gisele Bündchen's commitment to environmental causes is as strong as her impact on the fashion industry. As a globally recognized supermodel, she has used her platform to raise awareness about environmental issues, from deforestation to climate change. Throughout her career, Gisele has worked tirelessly to advocate for the planet, promoting sustainability and eco-friendly living in both her professional and personal life. Her deep connection to nature and her dedication to preserving the environment have made her a powerful voice in the movement for a greener, more sustainable world.

A Growing Awareness of Environmental Issues

Gisele's passion for environmental causes began early in her life. Growing up in Brazil, she developed a strong appreciation for nature and the importance of preserving the environment. This connection to the natural world influenced her understanding of the challenges facing the planet and motivated her to take action. Over the years, as she traveled around the globe for her modeling career, Gisele witnessed firsthand the impact of climate change and environmental destruction, which only deepened her commitment to sustainability.

As Gisele's career progressed, she began to use her influence and celebrity status to draw attention to critical environmental issues. She recognized the power of her platform in reaching millions of people and understood the responsibility that came with it. Instead of focusing solely on her modeling career, Gisele made it a priority to speak out on behalf of the planet, using her voice to highlight pressing environmental concerns.

One of the key aspects of Gisele's environmental activism is her focus on climate change. She has spoken extensively about the need for global action to address this issue, urging governments, businesses, and individuals to take responsibility for their environmental footprint. Gisele has participated in numerous campaigns and initiatives to raise awareness about climate change and its devastating effects, such as rising sea levels, extreme weather patterns, and loss of biodiversity. She has called for a shift toward renewable energy, cleaner transportation options, and the reduction of greenhouse gas emissions to help mitigate the effects of climate change.

Sustainability in Fashion and Beyond

In addition to raising awareness about climate change, Gisele has also focused on promoting sustainability within the fashion industry. As one of the most iconic supermodels of her generation, she has a unique ability to influence the choices of both consumers and brands. Throughout her career, Gisele has been vocal about the importance of sustainable fashion and the need for the industry to adopt more eco-friendly practices. She has advocated for brands to use sustainable materials, reduce waste, and adopt ethical production practices that minimize harm to the environment.

Gisele's dedication to sustainability extends beyond just words. She has put her beliefs into action. In 2011, she became the spokesperson for the environmental organization I'm Not a Plastic Bag, which encourages people to reduce their use of plastic and adopt more eco-friendly alternatives. She has also partnered with brands that prioritize sustainability, promoting environmentally conscious products in the fashion and beauty industries. One of the most notable examples of Gisele's commitment to sustainable fashion is her collaboration with the brand H&M, which focuses on producing clothing made from recycled materials. Through these partnerships, Gisele has worked to challenge the traditional practices of the fashion industry and encourage consumers to make more environmentally responsible choices.

Beyond fashion, Gisele has also been an advocate for sustainable living in all aspects of life. She has championed the use of renewable energy sources, such as solar power, and has spoken out about the importance of reducing carbon footprints. She practices what she preaches by using eco-friendly products, reducing waste, and supporting businesses that prioritize sustainability. Gisele's efforts to promote a more sustainable lifestyle have made her a role model for those who want to make a positive impact on the environment.

Conservation and Protection of Nature

One of Gisele's most significant contributions to environmental activism is her work in promoting conservation efforts, particularly in her home country of Brazil. The Amazon rainforest, often referred to as the "lungs of the Earth," has been a focal point of Gisele's environmental advocacy. She has spoken out about the importance of protecting the Amazon, not only because of its immense biodiversity but also because of its critical role in regulating the Earth's climate. Deforestation in the Amazon has led to increased greenhouse gas emissions, further exacerbating climate change. Gisele has used her platform to raise awareness about the importance of preserving this vital ecosystem.

In 2009, Gisele became a Goodwill Ambassador for the United Nations Environment Programme (UNEP), an organization dedicated to promoting sustainable development and protecting the environment. In this role, she has worked closely with UNEP to promote initiatives that focus on conservation, biodiversity, and the fight against climate change. She has also supported organizations such as the Rainforest Alliance and the Amazon Conservation Team, which work to protect the Amazon rainforest and other critical ecosystems around the world. Through her partnership with these organizations, Gisele has helped raise funds and visibility for conservation projects, emphasizing the importance of preserving nature for future generations.

Gisele's efforts to protect the environment are not limited to her advocacy work. She has also taken part in hands-on initiatives, such as tree-planting campaigns and environmental cleanup efforts. She has actively participated in projects aimed at restoring degraded lands and protecting endangered species, working alongside experts and organizations to ensure that her contributions have a meaningful and lasting impact.

Raising Awareness and Inspiring Change

As a global icon, Gisele has the unique ability to reach millions of people around the world. Through her environmental activism, she has become a powerful voice for change, inspiring others to take action and make a difference. She has used her visibility to educate her followers about the importance of environmental protection, encouraging them to adopt sustainable practices in their daily lives. Whether it's reducing plastic waste, supporting eco-friendly businesses, or taking steps to minimize their carbon footprint, Gisele has empowered her audience to become more environmentally conscious.

Through social media, interviews, and public appearances, Gisele continues to raise awareness about environmental issues, using her platform to educate and inspire. She has shared her personal experiences with sustainability, offering tips and advice on how individuals can make a positive impact on the environment. Her message is clear: every small action counts, and collectively, these actions can create a significant difference in the fight against climate change.

Gisele's commitment to the environment has earned her recognition and respect in the world of environmental activism. She has been honored for her efforts to raise awareness about climate change and promote sustainability, receiving awards from environmental organizations and global leaders. Her dedication to the planet has made her a respected figure in both the fashion industry and the environmental movement, and her influence continues to grow.

A Lasting Legacy of Environmental Advocacy

Gisele's environmental activism is a testament to her commitment to making a positive impact on the planet. She has proven that being a successful supermodel doesn't mean one cannot be a force for change in the world. Through her advocacy work, her dedication to sustainability, and her efforts to raise awareness about climate change, Gisele has made a lasting contribution to the environmental movement.

As the world continues to face environmental challenges, Gisele's voice remains an important one in the fight for a more sustainable future. Her work has inspired countless individuals, businesses, and organizations to take action and make choices that are better for the planet. Gisele Bündchen's commitment to environmental activism will continue to shape the conversation around climate change and sustainability for years to come, ensuring that her legacy extends far beyond the fashion world.

CHAPTER 9: Love and Family-Personal Life in the Spotlight

Gisele Bündchen's life has always been in the spotlight, not just because of her career as one of the world's most famous supermodels but also because of her relationships. Her marriage to football superstar Tom Brady, her experience with motherhood, and the way she balances her family life with her career have all played significant roles in shaping her public persona. While Gisele has been open about many aspects of her life, she has also managed to maintain a level of privacy, sharing only what feels right for her and her loved ones.

The Beginning of a Love Story: Meeting Tom Brady

One of the most talked-about relationships in the world of celebrities has been Gisele's marriage to NFL quarterback Tom Brady. The two first met in 2006, through mutual friends, and immediately hit it off. However, their relationship did not develop into something serious right away. Gisele, who had just come out of a long-term relationship, was not initially looking for love. She was focused on her career and the various personal and professional goals she had set for herself.

At first, Gisele had reservations about Tom, who, despite being a famous football player, was going through some struggles in his own life. Tom had recently gone through a breakup and was dealing with the pressure of being in the public eye. However, as they spent more time together, Gisele realized that there was something special about him. Tom, for his part, was drawn to Gisele's down-to-earth nature, beauty, and intelligence.

Their relationship grew quickly, and by 2009, they were married in a small, private ceremony in Santa Monica, California. This union was not just the coming together of two famous figures, but it was the start of a strong partnership built on trust, mutual respect, and shared values. Over the years, their relationship has become one of the most admired in Hollywood, often seen as a model of love, dedication, and family values.

Motherhood: A New Chapter in Gisele's Life

For Gisele, becoming a mother was one of the most transformative experiences of her life. In 2009, just a few months after her wedding to Tom, Gisele became a stepmother to his son, John Edward Thomas Moynahan, from his previous relationship with actress Bridget Moynahan. Though it was an adjustment to take on the role of a stepmother, Gisele embraced it wholeheartedly, dedicating herself to making sure that her new family blended well together. She has often spoken about how her bond with John is very special, and she has always treated him with the same love and care that she gives her biological children.

In December 2009, Gisele and Tom welcomed their first child together, a son named Benjamin Rein Brady. Gisele's experience with motherhood took on new dimensions as she navigated the challenges of balancing her successful modeling career with the needs of her growing family. As a mother, Gisele has emphasized the importance of family time, healthy living, and maintaining a strong emotional connection with her children.

She has always sought to raise her children with a sense of responsibility and grounded values. Gisele has shared how she wants her children to appreciate nature, understand the importance of kindness, and develop a strong sense of empathy. For her, family life is about creating an environment where her children feel loved, safe, and free to grow into their best selves.

In 2012, Gisele and Tom expanded their family further with the birth of their daughter, Vivian Lake Brady. As a mother of two, Gisele found herself constantly juggling the demands of motherhood with her high-profile career. Despite her busy schedule, she has always prioritized spending quality time with her family. Gisele has described how her family life is at the heart of everything she does, and she strives to find a balance that allows her to give her children the attention they need while still pursuing her professional ambitions.

Balancing Family and Career- The Art of Prioritization

Gisele's ability to balance her family life with her demanding career has been one of the key reasons for her enduring success. As a top model, she has worked with some of the biggest brands and walked in the most prestigious fashion shows. Yet, she has always managed to keep her family as her number one priority. For Gisele, family comes before everything else, and she has often spoken about the importance of being present for her children and her husband.

Over the years, Gisele has taken breaks from her modeling career to focus on her family. She has been open about the fact that she doesn't want to work nonstop, but instead seeks to find a healthy balance. She has said that the key to balancing family and career is to listen to her heart and make choices based on what feels right at the time. This approach has allowed her to continue working in the industry while also being a devoted wife and mother.

Gisele has also praised Tom for being supportive of her career and the demands it entails. Their partnership has always been one of equal respect, with both of them recognizing the importance of each other's work and ambitions. Tom, too, has made sacrifices to ensure that he is present for his family. As a professional athlete with a demanding schedule, he has often adjusted his commitments to prioritize family life, making time for Gisele and their children whenever possible.

The couple has always been private about their family life, preferring to keep their moments out of the public eye as much as possible. This decision has allowed them to protect their family and provide their children with a stable environment, away from the pressures of fame.

The Role of Gisele's Family in Shaping Her Identity

While Gisele has always been recognized as one of the world's most successful models, her family life has been integral to her sense of identity. The support she receives from her husband and children has been a foundation upon which she has built her career. Gisele has shared how important it is for her to maintain a close-knit family unit, where love, respect, and support are central.

She has also acknowledged that being a mother and wife has taught her valuable life lessons that she applies to her work. The experience of raising children has made her more patient, grounded, and focused. It has reminded her of the importance of leading with kindness and compassion, both at home and in her professional life.

Through her relationship with Tom and her role as a mother, Gisele has learned to prioritize what truly matters family, love, and personal happiness. This approach has not only helped her navigate the challenges of fame but has also allowed her to be an inspiration to others who seek to balance family life with their careers.

A Family-Oriented Life in the Public Eye

Throughout her career, Gisele has made it clear that her family life is of utmost importance. Her relationship with Tom Brady, her role as a stepmother and mother, and her ability to juggle family and career have all been significant factors in shaping her public image. Despite the pressures that come with being in the public eye, Gisele has remained committed to creating a private, loving home for her family. Through her example, she has shown that it is possible to maintain a successful career while nurturing the bonds that truly matter.

CHAPTER 10: THE BUSINESS MOGUL -A GISELE AS AN ENTREPRENEUR

Gisele Bündchen's career has always been defined by more than just her modeling prowess. As one of the highest-paid supermodels in the world, Gisele has skillfully leveraged her fame and influence to build a thriving empire that extends far beyond the runway. Through her entrepreneurial ventures, she has established herself not only as a global fashion icon but also as a savvy businesswoman with a keen sense for opportunities.

Skincare Line-A Personal Commitment to Health and Wellness

One of Gisele's most notable business ventures is her skincare line, Seja. Launched in 2018, the line is built around Gisele's passion for sustainability and natural beauty. Inspired by her skincare routine and commitment to using non-toxic products, Seja aims to promote healthy, radiant skin using eco-friendly, organic ingredients. The brand focuses on environmentally conscious packaging and supports ethical sourcing of its components, aligning with Gisele's advocacy for a greener planet.

What makes Seja unique is the personal touch Gisele brings to it. With her extensive experience in the beauty and fashion industries, she carefully curated the products to meet the demands of a wide audience. Seja's range includes everything from moisturizers and cleansers to serums and sunscreens. Each product is designed to promote skin wellness, focusing on hydration, anti-aging, and nourishment. The emphasis is on simple, clean beauty that avoids harsh chemicals while still delivering visible results.

Gisele's investment in Seja is more than just a commercial endeavor. It reflects her personal belief in taking care of the body and using products that align with her values. She regularly promotes the brand through her social media channels, where her large following connects with her message of authenticity and self-care.

Investments: Strategic Choices for Long-Term Success

In addition to her beauty brand, Gisele has made several smart investments in various industries, demonstrating her sharp business acumen. Over the years, she has been involved in real estate ventures, startups, and tech companies, showing her versatility as an investor.

One of her most notable investments is in the wellness and eco-friendly sectors. She has put money into companies that focus on sustainability and the environment, such as the sustainable fashion brand H&M Conscious and

Patagonia, a company known for its environmentally responsible practices. These investments align with Gisele's values of promoting a healthier planet and supporting businesses that share her passion for sustainability.

Moreover, Gisele has shown interest in the wellness industry, investing in startups that promote healthy living and mindfulness. By partnering with companies that focus on organic, clean products, she not only diversifies her portfolio but also ensures her investments are aligned with her own lifestyle choices.

Her approach to investing is guided by her desire to make a positive impact on the world while securing long-term financial growth. Gisele's investment strategies have proven successful, cementing her position as a financially savvy entrepreneur who is both mindful of the world and focused on building wealth.

Branding Partnerships-A Powerful Presence in the Business World

Gisele's role as a brand ambassador and her various partnerships with top companies are another cornerstone of her business empire. Over the years, she has collaborated with major global brands, leveraging her image and influence to create lucrative deals. These partnerships have solidified her as a leading figure in the world of branding, where her credibility and presence elevate the companies she works with.

One of Gisele's most significant partnerships has been with the luxury fashion brand Louis Vuitton, where she became the face of several successful ad campaigns. Her work with Louis Vuitton catapulted her into the realm of high fashion and luxury branding, where she represented not just the brand's clothes, but its core values of elegance, sophistication, and timeless beauty.

Additionally, Gisele has worked with global beauty and health brands, such as Pantene and Chanel, where she further cemented her status as a beauty icon. These partnerships allowed her to diversify her portfolio and expand her reach to different industries, from hair care to fragrances.

Her brand collaborations also include the renowned shoe company Ipanema, where she created a line of sandals. This venture allowed Gisele to tap into the casual, stylish footwear market, further diversifying her business interests. Her partnership with Ipanema was a natural fit, as it aligned with her Brazilian roots and her focus on comfort and fashion.

The success of these partnerships lies not only in Gisele's global popularity but also in her ability to connect with consumers on a personal level. Her genuine endorsement of the products she represents is a significant factor in their success. Whether she's promoting a fashion brand, a beauty product, or an eco-friendly initiative, Gisele's credibility and authenticity shine through, making her an incredibly valuable asset to companies looking to boost their image.

A Vision for the Future: Expanding the Brand

Looking ahead, Gisele continues to focus on expanding her business ventures. Her commitment to sustainability and social responsibility has led her to explore more eco-conscious initiatives, and she plans to continue to invest in companies that prioritize the environment and health. With her diverse range of businesses, Gisele is not just a supermodel but a formidable entrepreneur, building an empire that is grounded in her values of self-care, sustainability, and social impact.

In the years to come, Gisele's brand will likely expand even further, with new business ventures and collaborations. She has proven time and time again that her entrepreneurial spirit goes beyond her career as a model. By carefully selecting investments, promoting ethical products, and aligning with like-minded companies, Gisele has carved a path for herself as a successful and forward-thinking business mogul. Her ability to remain authentic while simultaneously growing her brand is a testament to her enduring appeal and business acumen.

Gisele Bündchen's entrepreneurial journey showcases her deep understanding of the business world. Through her skincare line, strategic investments, and impactful brand partnerships, she has built a diverse and lucrative business empire that extends her influence far beyond the world of modeling.

CHAPTER 11: CULTURAL ICON-THE LASTING INFLUENCE OF GISELE BUNDCHEN

Gisele Bündchen is much more than a supermodel; she has become a cultural icon whose influence spans far beyond the fashion industry. Her journey from a small town in Brazil to the global stage has been marked by her ability to connect with people on a deeper level, shaping trends, influencing pop culture, and inspiring younger generations. Gisele's impact is felt in the way she has redefined beauty standards, become a role model, and left a lasting mark on the world in various fields.

Redefining Beauty Standards: A New Ideal

Gisele's most significant contribution to popular culture is her role in challenging and reshaping beauty standards. When Gisele entered the fashion industry, the dominant beauty ideal was that of the ultra-thin model. However, Gisele's body type, which was more athletic and curvaceous, defied the conventional norms and resonated with a broader audience. She became the face of a new, healthier, and more inclusive vision of beauty. Her natural look, with a glowing tan, sun-kissed hair, and radiant skin, presented a more attainable and down-to-earth ideal.

Her success helped redefine the image of the supermodel, where beauty was no longer limited to one body type. This change had a ripple effect across the fashion industry, influencing how other models were cast and how beauty was portrayed in advertising, magazine covers, and runway shows. Gisele's influence paved the way for a more diverse representation of beauty, one that included different body types, skin tones, and features. Today, many models have followed in her footsteps, embracing more natural and diverse representations of beauty.

A Symbol of Empowerment and Confidence

Beyond her physical appearance, Gisele has also become a symbol of empowerment. As one of the highest-paid models in the world, she broke barriers and proved that women could achieve financial independence and success on their terms. Her career exemplified the power of self-confidence, and she encouraged women to embrace their uniqueness and follow their paths. Gisele has often spoken about the importance of self-love, resilience, and staying true to oneself, messages that resonated with millions of young women worldwide.

Her impact is not just about appearance but about how she carries herself. Gisele's confidence, poise, and strength have been an inspiration to many, teaching them that true beauty comes from within. Her journey has shown that success doesn't require conforming to someone else's standards but rather embracing one's individuality and power. She continues to be a voice for empowerment, inspiring women to lead with confidence and authenticity.

Influence on Fashion Trends-Setting the Standard

As a fashion icon, Gisele has played an instrumental role in setting trends and influencing the way people approach style. From her signature tousled beach waves to her effortless, yet chic, fashion sense, Gisele's style has always been admired by fashion enthusiasts worldwide. She became the face of countless high-fashion brands, and her runway presence was a hallmark of top-tier fashion shows, setting trends that were copied by millions.

What made Gisele's influence unique is her ability to balance luxury fashion with more casual, accessible looks. She was just as comfortable in a glamorous gown on the runway as she was in a pair of jeans and a simple t-shirt, representing the idea that style is about personal expression rather than following rigid rules. Her effortlessly chic aesthetic resonated with people who wanted to incorporate high-fashion elements into their everyday wardrobe without sacrificing comfort.

Furthermore, Gisele's collaboration with brands such as Chanel, Louis Vuitton, and Balenciaga set a precedent for how models could influence trends. Her work with these brands not only elevated their status but also made their designs more widely accessible to consumers who wanted to emulate her style. Gisele's ability to make fashion feel attainable while maintaining its aspirational quality has been a key part of her influence on global fashion trends.

A Role Model for Younger Generations

Gisele's impact on younger generations is profound, especially in how she has navigated the pressures of fame and the modeling industry. She has been open about her struggles with body image, self-doubt, and the challenges of maintaining a public persona. By sharing these experiences, Gisele has become a relatable figure for young people facing similar issues. She has shown that even the most successful individuals face challenges, and it's okay to be vulnerable and imperfect.

Her messages of self-care, balance, and prioritizing mental health have become especially important in today's world, where social media often presents an unrealistic standard of perfection. Through her interviews, books, and social media platforms, Gisele has emphasized the importance of taking care of one's emotional and mental well-being, in addition to physical health. She frequently advocates for slowing down, spending time in nature, and reconnecting with what truly matters, offering a refreshing contrast to the often fast-paced, appearance-driven culture of the modern world.

In this sense, Gisele has become more than just a fashion icon; she is a mentor and role model for young people who look up to her not just for her looks but for her values. Her life and career show that true success is about more than external appearances .it's about living with integrity, being kind, and nurturing one's well-being.

Philanthropy and Advocacy-Using Fame for Good

Gisele's influence extends into philanthropy and activism, where she has used her platform to advocate for important causes, particularly environmental sustainability. Through her advocacy for climate change awareness, Gisele has brought attention to issues that affect the planet and its future. Her efforts to promote eco-friendly products, sustainable practices, and climate action align with her desire to leave a positive legacy beyond the fashion industry.

She has been involved in several environmental initiatives, working with organizations like the United Nations Environment Programme (UNEP) to promote green living and sustainable development. Her commitment to sustainability is reflected in her business ventures as well, such as her eco-friendly skincare line, which emphasizes the importance of conscious consumption. Gisele's dedication to environmental causes has inspired many of her fans and followers to make more mindful choices about the products they buy and the impact they have on the world.

A Timeless Cultural Force

Gisele Bündchen's lasting influence as a cultural icon is evident in the way she has shaped fashion, beauty, and the way society views confidence and empowerment. From redefining beauty standards to being a role model for younger generations, Gisele's impact is far-reaching. She continues to inspire millions not only through her career but also through her advocacy, personal beliefs, and the legacy she continues to build. As she evolves and continues to inspire, her influence will undoubtedly be felt for generations to come. Gisele is more than a supermodel; she is a cultural force whose impact extends far beyond the runway.

CHAPTER 12: OVERCOMING OBSTACLES- CHALLENGES AND RESILIENCE

Gisele Bündchen's journey to becoming one of the most successful supermodels in the world has not been without its obstacles. Behind her glamorous career and widespread success, Gisele has faced a range of personal and professional challenges. Yet, through each struggle, she has shown remarkable resilience. Her ability to navigate these hardships has not only shaped her career but has also made her a source of inspiration to many who look up to her.

Early Struggles in the Modeling Industry

When Gisele first entered the modeling world, she faced significant challenges. At 14, she was discovered in São Paulo, Brazil, and quickly signed by a modeling agency. However, her early years in the industry were not easy. Initially, Gisele struggled to fit into the high-fashion world's narrow standards. She didn't have the slender, waif-like frame that was popular in the 1990s, which led to initial rejections from major fashion houses. During her first few years as a model, Gisele was often told that she was too curvy or too tall to succeed in the competitive industry.

This early rejection was a difficult period for her. It could have discouraged anyone, but Gisele remained determined to prove herself.

Rather than conform to the industry's rigid standards, she embraced her natural body and distinctive look, which set her apart from other models. Over time, her unique features began to shine, and she was able to secure more work, eventually becoming one of the most in-demand models in the world.

Facing Body Image Pressures

As a supermodel, Gisele was constantly in the public eye, and the pressure to maintain a perfect appearance was immense. In an industry where weight, height, and body shape are scrutinized, Gisele faced the challenge of balancing her physical health with her professional expectations. Like many models, she was often expected to maintain a certain weight and physique to fit into the clothes designed by high-fashion designers. This pressure led her to struggle with body image issues, especially early in her career.

At one point, Gisele even admitted to feeling insecure about her body, especially when she compared herself to other, often thinner models. She shared in interviews how difficult it was to see herself as "good enough" given the industry's emphasis on achieving perfection. However, rather than allowing these insecurities to overwhelm her, Gisele took a different approach. She focused on staying healthy, and over time, she learned to embrace her body as it was. Gisele's decision to stop trying to conform to one narrow standard of beauty and instead focus on her well-being was a turning point in her personal growth. She realized that self-love and acceptance were the keys to her mental and emotional resilience, and this belief became central to her career and life.

Public Scrutiny and Negative Media Attention

As a global superstar, Gisele has also had to contend with the constant scrutiny of the media. While fame brought her many opportunities, it also meant being the subject of criticism and gossip. From speculation about her personal life to harsh judgments about her appearance, the media attention was often intrusive and negative. One of the most intense periods of public scrutiny came during her marriage to NFL superstar Tom Brady. The couple's every move was heavily reported on, and tabloids frequently speculated on their relationship, health, and family matters.

This constant media attention could have been overwhelming for anyone, but Gisele faced it with quiet strength. Instead of reacting defensively, she chose to focus on what truly mattered to her—her family, her career, and her values. She learned to ignore the noise and keep her personal life as private as possible, giving her the space to cultivate a balanced and grounded life despite the public pressure. Gisele has often stated that the key to dealing with negative media attention was learning to prioritize her well-being over the opinions of others.

Overcoming Career Doubts and Burnout

Throughout her career, Gisele faced moments of doubt and burnout, especially after years of grueling schedules and constant travel. While many viewed her as the pinnacle of success, Gisele went through periods of questioning her place in the industry. At one point, she considered stepping away from modeling to focus on other pursuits. She felt disconnected from her true self and longed for a sense of peace and fulfillment outside of the fast-paced, high-pressure world of fashion.

During this period of uncertainty, Gisele took time off to focus on herself. She began meditating, practicing yoga, and reconnecting with nature, all of which helped her regain a sense of balance. By taking care of her mental and emotional health, she found the strength to continue her career while aligning it with her values. Gisele's ability to recognize when she needed to slow down and re-evaluate her priorities allowed her to stay true to her passions and ultimately return to the industry with renewed purpose.

Balancing Family and Career

Another significant challenge Gisele faced was the balancing act between her professional ambitions and her personal life. After marrying Tom Brady and having children, she had to navigate the demands of a high-profile career while being a mother and wife. Juggling the responsibilities of family life with the pressures of maintaining a successful modeling career was no easy feat, and Gisele often spoke about the difficulty of finding that balance.

She has been open about her struggles with balancing these two aspects of her life, noting that it wasn't always easy to prioritize her family while also maintaining her career. But through time management, support from her family, and a firm commitment to her values, Gisele found a way to make it work. She decided to take on fewer professional commitments to spend more time with her children, demonstrating her resilience in maintaining a healthy work-life balance.

Personal Growth and Empowerment

Through these many challenges, Gisele has emerged stronger and more empowered. Her personal growth over the years has been shaped by the struggles she faced and the resilience she developed in overcoming them. She has learned to embrace imperfections, ignore external pressures, and focus on the things that bring her joy and peace. These lessons have become central to her identity, and today, Gisele is not only a successful businesswoman and philanthropist but also a role model for anyone facing obstacles in their own lives.

Gisele's journey shows that resilience is not about avoiding challenges, but about facing them with grace and perseverance. She has shown that it is possible to overcome adversity, whether it be career setbacks, body image pressures, or personal doubts, and emerge stronger on the other side. Her story continues to inspire people worldwide, proving that even in the face of difficulties, resilience can lead to growth, success, and fulfillment.

CHAPTER 13: PHILANTROPY-GIVING BACK TO THE WORLD

Gisele Bündchen is not only known for her incredible career as a supermodel but also for her dedication to philanthropy. Throughout her life, she has used her platform to raise awareness and support a variety of charitable causes. Whether advocating for environmental sustainability, supporting underprivileged communities, or promoting mental health awareness, Gisele has shown that true success is about making a positive impact in the world. Her commitment to giving back is deeply ingrained in her values, and she continuously strives to create social change through her charitable efforts.

Environmental Advocacy- A Strong Commitment to Sustainability

One of Gisele's most prominent philanthropic efforts is her dedication to environmental sustainability. She has long been an advocate for protecting the planet and combating climate change, using her fame to bring attention to the urgent need for environmental action. Gisele has worked with a range of environmental organizations, including the United Nations Environment Programme (UNEP), to raise awareness about issues such as deforestation, pollution, and the impact of climate change on vulnerable communities.

Gisele's advocacy is not just limited to raising awareness but extends to promoting sustainable practices in her personal and professional life. For example, she has made conscious choices to live a more eco-friendly lifestyle, from eating a plant-based diet to reducing her carbon footprint. She also launched her line of eco-friendly skincare products, which emphasizes natural ingredients and sustainable packaging. Gisele believes that small, mindful changes can have a big impact on the planet, and she encourages others to make environmentally conscious choices in their daily lives as well.

Through her involvement with various environmental causes, Gisele has been able to use her platform to amplify the voices of those working to protect the earth. She is a vocal advocate for the preservation of the Amazon rainforest, a region close to her heart due to her Brazilian roots. She actively supports initiatives aimed at preserving this vital ecosystem and the indigenous communities that rely on it. Gisele's philanthropic efforts in environmentalism highlight her belief that the planet's future is everyone's responsibility.

Supporting Underprivileged Communities- Making a Difference Locally and Globally

In addition to her environmental work, Gisele is deeply committed to supporting underprivileged communities around the world. She believes in using her resources to uplift those who are less fortunate and to provide them with the tools they need to improve their lives. Gisele has worked with several organizations that focus on education, poverty alleviation, and healthcare for marginalized groups.

One of the causes Gisele is particularly passionate about is education. She understands the transformative power of education in breaking the cycle of poverty, and she has supported numerous programs that provide young people with access to quality education. Gisele has been involved with the Rainforest Alliance, which works to improve the lives of rural communities in the Amazon by supporting sustainable livelihoods and education. She has also donated to causes that provide children with access to better healthcare and educational opportunities, believing that empowering the next generation is key to creating long-term change.

Gisele has also used her own experiences as a role model to inspire young people to pursue their dreams, regardless of their background or circumstances. She often speaks about the importance of resilience and determination, encouraging young people to take control of their futures. Her story of rising from humble beginnings in Brazil to become a global icon serves as a powerful reminder that anyone, no matter their origins, can achieve greatness.

Mental Health Advocacy-A Personal Mission

Beyond her work in environmental sustainability and supporting underprivileged communities, Gisele is also passionate about raising awareness for mental health issues. She has been open about her struggles with anxiety and stress, sharing how she has learned to manage her mental health through meditation, yoga, and self-care practices. Gisele's honesty about her mental health challenges has helped reduce the stigma around these issues, especially in the fashion industry, where pressure and stress are often overlooked.

In addition to advocating for mental health awareness, Gisele has also been involved in initiatives that aim to support mental health care and provide resources for those in need. She works with organizations that focus on providing psychological support to individuals and communities affected by trauma, including children in conflict zones and people who have experienced natural disasters. Gisele believes that mental health is just as important as physical health and that everyone deserves access to the care and resources they need to lead fulfilling lives.

Gisele's efforts in promoting mental health have been especially impactful in the way they challenge societal norms and encourage individuals to prioritize their well-being. She has often spoken out about the pressures of fame and the unrealistic expectations placed on individuals in the public eye, using her own experiences to advocate for a healthier approach to life. By encouraging others to seek help and embrace self-care, Gisele has helped foster a more open and compassionate conversation about mental health in society.

Creating Long-Term Social Change-Empowering Future Generations

For Gisele, philanthropy is not just about making temporary donations; it's about creating long-term social change that will benefit future generations. One of the ways she has done this is through her active involvement in organizations that focus on creating sustainable, community-driven solutions to social problems. Gisele has supported initiatives that teach skills and offer resources to help individuals become self-sufficient, empowering them to take control of their futures.

Through her work with organizations like the Icelandic Glacial Initiative, Gisele has championed the importance of clean water access for all. She has advocated for the responsible management of water resources, especially in underdeveloped regions, where access to clean drinking water is limited. Gisele believes that ensuring clean water is available to everyone is fundamental to health, education, and economic development. By addressing these fundamental issues, Gisele has helped create a foundation for lasting social change.

Gisele is involved with organizations that help women and children gain access to resources, education, and economic opportunities. She has supported campaigns that focus on ending child labor, promoting gender equality, and ensuring that women have access to healthcare and education. Gisele's work in these areas reflects her belief that empowering women and children is key to breaking the cycle of poverty and creating a more equitable world.

A Legacy of Giving Back

Gisele Bündchen's philanthropic efforts have made a significant and lasting impact on the world. Whether she's advocating for environmental sustainability, supporting underprivileged communities, or raising awareness for mental health, Gisele has shown that giving back is not just about financial contributions but about dedicating time, resources, and energy to causes that truly matter. Her ongoing commitment to creating positive social change continues to inspire millions, and her legacy as a philanthropist is a testament to the power of using one's platform for good. Gisele's work reminds us all that true success is not only measured by personal achievements but also by how we contribute to improving the world around us.

CHAPTER 14: LEGACY OF A SUPERMODEL- GISELE'S ENDURING INFLUENCE

Gisele Bündchen is more than just a supermodel; she is a symbol of transformation, success, and resilience in the fashion world and beyond. Over the years, Gisele has become a defining figure in the modeling industry and a global icon whose influence extends far beyond the runway. Her journey from a small town in Brazil to one of the highest-paid and most recognized models in the world has left an indelible mark on both the fashion industry and popular culture. As her career continues to evolve, Gisele's legacy as a pioneering force in fashion and as a role model remains a powerful inspiration for future generations.

Breaking Barriers in the Fashion Industry

Gisele's impact on the fashion industry is immeasurable. When she first entered the modeling world in the late 1990s, the industry was dominated by a different type of beauty lean, and often, almost skeletal. At the time, models with waif-like figures, like Kate Moss, were the standard of beauty. Gisele, however, represented a shift from that aesthetic. With her tall, athletic frame and striking curves, she brought a new type of beauty into the spotlight. Her presence on the runway and in magazines marked the beginning of a new era in fashion, where diversity in body types and beauty standards began to take root.

Gisele's rise to fame coincided with the end of the "supermodel era" and the rise of a new, more inclusive age in fashion. She was one of the first models to break the traditional mold, and her success helped to challenge the industry's narrow definitions of beauty. Her distinctive look and powerful runway presence made her one of the most sought-after models of her time. Gisele's influence helped pave the way for a more diverse representation of beauty in the fashion world, encouraging designers, photographers, and brands to think more inclusively when it came to casting models.

Her ability to blend elegance with strength and vulnerability made her a favorite of some of the most respected designers, from Alexander McQueen to Dolce & Gabbana. She redefined what it meant to be a "model," as she was not only a face, but a force an embodiment of both beauty and strength. Gisele showed the fashion world that models could be more than just pretty faces they could be powerful women who could change the industry through their talent and influence.

The Victoria's Secret Era and Global Recognition

One of the most significant chapters in Gisele's career was her association with Victoria's Secret. When she became a Victoria's Secret Angel in 2000, she entered into one of the most iconic relationships between a model and a brand. Her role as an Angel skyrocketed her visibility and solidified her status as one of the world's most famous supermodels. The Victoria's Secret fashion shows, which featured Gisele in her prime, became global spectacles watched by millions. Gisele was the face of the brand during its most successful years, and her appearances helped define the glamour and appeal of Victoria's Secret, bringing the company to international prominence.

Her time as an Angel was a defining moment in her career. Gisele's presence on the runway at the Victoria's Secret Fashion Show made her a household name, and her beauty, confidence, and charisma were key factors in the company's rise to global dominance. For years, she was the star of the show, walking in iconic lingerie fashion shows that became synonymous with luxury and allure. As the brand's top model, Gisele was instrumental in shaping the image of Victoria's Secret, and her success within the company helped her become a global icon, solidifying her position in the history of fashion.

However, even beyond her work with Victoria's Secret, Gisele's influence in the fashion world became undeniable. Her campaigns with major luxury brands, such as Chanel, Louis Vuitton, and Versace, set the standard for models in the 21st century. Gisele brought a rare combination of beauty, poise, and personality to every campaign, becoming the face of high-end fashion and contributing to a broader shift in the fashion world toward models who embodied both strength and sophistication.

A Business Mogul with Vision

Gisele's influence is not confined to the runway. She has also made a name for herself as a successful entrepreneur and businesswoman. Her ventures outside of modeling, including her skincare line and environmental initiatives, are central to her legacy. By branching out into business, Gisele proved that she was not just a pretty face but a savvy entrepreneur with vision and determination. Her ability to leverage her fame to build a brand around her personal values, sustainability, wellness, and beauty. Further solidified her as a figure who was not simply a product of the fashion industry, but a true business mogul in her own right.

Her skincare line, Sejaa, for example, emphasizes the use of natural ingredients and environmentally responsible practices. Through this line, Gisele has been able to promote her belief in the importance of self-care and environmental sustainability. This venture reflects her broader philosophy of caring for both one's body and the planet. Gisele's move into business not only diversified her career but also cemented her role as an influential figure in both the fashion and business worlds.

Moreover, her investments in various startups and branding partnerships reflect her foresight as a businesswoman. Gisele has worked with companies that align with her values, whether in beauty, lifestyle, or environmental causes. Her smart decisions have made her an example of how to build a lasting legacy beyond the traditional career path of a model.

A Global Icon: Beyond Fashion

Gisele's legacy extends beyond the world of fashion. She has become a global icon whose influence touches various aspects of culture and society. As one of the most recognizable faces in the world, Gisele's impact transcends her career as a model. She is an active voice in global conversations on climate change, women's rights, and mental health, using her platform to advocate for causes that matter to her.

Her philanthropy, in particular, has been a significant aspect of her global influence. Gisele has long been dedicated to environmental causes, and she continues to work with organizations such as the United Nations

Environment Programme (UNEP) to raise awareness about sustainability and the need to protect the planet. Through her advocacy and actions, Gisele has become a role model for others who seek to use their fame for positive change. Her charitable work has made her a leader in the fight for social and environmental justice, and her efforts have inspired others to get involved and make a difference.

 Gisele's influence extends to the way she represents women in the public eye. She has challenged traditional beauty standards and encouraged self-acceptance. As a mother, wife, and businesswoman, Gisele embodies the modern woman who balances personal and professional ambitions while remaining true to her values. Her story serves as an inspiration to millions, showing that it is possible to achieve success while maintaining authenticity and integrity.

The Enduring Influence of Gisele Bündchen

As Gisele continues to evolve in her career and personal life, her legacy remains an indelible part of the fashion world and global culture. From her groundbreaking work in the modeling industry to her entrepreneurial success and philanthropic contributions, Gisele has left a lasting impact on how we view beauty, success, and responsibility. Her ability to break barriers, redefine beauty standards, and influence change has solidified her place as one of the most significant figures in fashion history.

Gisele's legacy is not just about her achievements, but about how she has used her platform to inspire others, give back to the world, and remain authentic in the face of fame. She is a pioneering force whose influence will continue to be felt for years to come, both within the fashion industry and across the globe. Her impact is a reminder that true greatness is measured not just by personal success, but by how we uplift others and contribute to the world around us.

CONCLUSION

Gisele Bündchen - A Supermodel's Journey to
Stardom

Gisele Bündchen's story is one of remarkable
transformation and undeniable influence. From
her humble beginnings in a small town in Brazil
to becoming one of the most recognized and
successful supermodels in the world, her journey
has been nothing short of inspiring. She didn't
just conform to the expectations of the modeling
industry; she reshaped them, challenging beauty
standards and proving that strength, confidence,
and individuality could redefine what it meant to
be a model.

Through her hard work, perseverance, and dedication, Gisele broke through barriers, not only achieving incredible success on the runway but also becoming a global icon and business mogul. Her collaborations with major brands, her ventures into entrepreneurship, and her advocacy for environmental and social causes all reflect her multidimensional impact on the world. But beyond her professional achievements, Gisele's ability to balance fame with family, charity, and her values has shown the world that success isn't just about career accomplishments. It's about making a positive difference and staying true to oneself.

Her legacy is one of resilience, empowerment, and giving back. Whether she's speaking out for the planet, supporting women's rights, or raising awareness for mental health, Gisele has used her platform to promote meaningful change. As a philanthropist and a role model, she has inspired countless individuals to pursue their passions and embrace their unique journey, no matter the obstacles.

Gisele Bündchen's path to stardom is not just a tale of a supermodel. It's a testament to the power of determination, kindness, and authenticity. Her story continues to inspire people around the world, reminding us that with hard work, compassion, and a strong sense of purpose, anyone can achieve greatness and leave a lasting legacy.

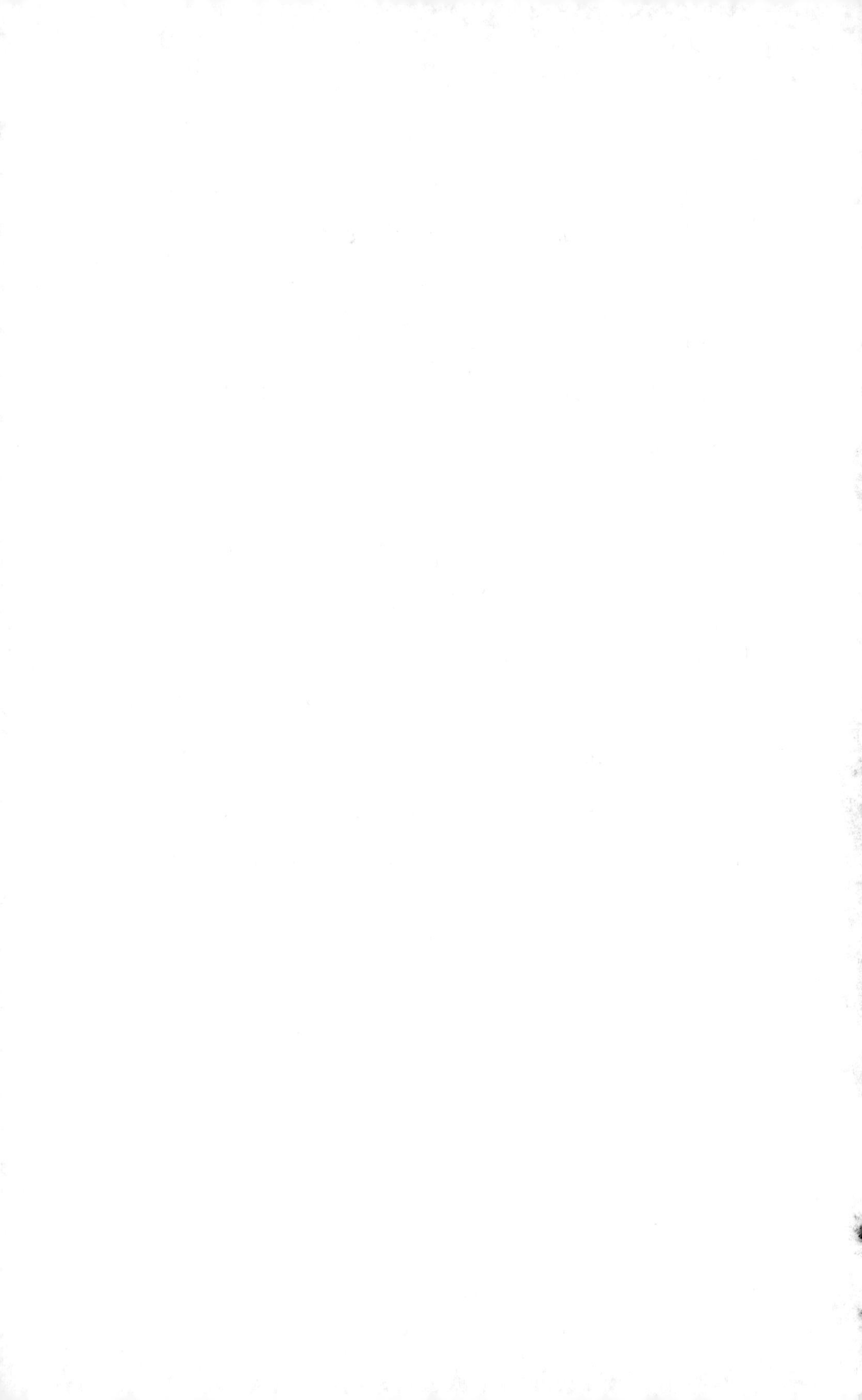